MSM - THE MISSING LINK TO OPTIMAL HEALTH

PETER CARL SIMONS

Made with ❤ on the Notion Press Platform
www.notionpress.com

Contents

Sulfur is an important mineral nutrient, and it is essential for the body of a person. MSM is the key element that will complete the missing link to the optimal health of a person. It is an extremely vital element but sometimes overshadowed by the potassium, nitrogen, and phosphorus. When understanding the use of sulfur and its need for the body, it is also significant to know that how the sulfur has an important and central role in the soil condition, the growth of the plants and the human health. It is an important part that needs to be discussed as the utilization of sulfur is important for getting the optimized crop quality and yield. Additionally, it must be focused that when the sulfur is included in the Methionine and cysteine in the plants, it comes out with a straight effect on the nutritional value of the livestock feeds as well as the human food. The aim of this book has been considered important as it will give information about the MSM and how it will fill the missing link to the optimal health. The sulfur is important and missing in the soil, plants, and nutrition.

The books are very important when they come to provide the information to the people about the health issues. The health learning books are usually written to give the most interesting as well as the useful knowledge and information about the health of a person. This information is used to improve the health of a person that tells that what the body needs to maintain good health as well as the missing link to the optimal health will be filled.

The diseases are not everything. The good health is usually considered without the issues of any diseases. It is not a point that must be considered. The people think that the person who does not have any disease is having good health. This type of negative disease-oriented thinking must be avoided to put emphasis on the points that help a person to stay healthy.

The health of a person is very important and to reach the optimal health, the person must think of supplying the essential nutrients and elements that the body requires but on the daily basis. When the body of a person is given all the essential and vital nutrients, the diseases will no longer be affecting, but once the body does not get the desired nutrients, the diseases will be resulting to cause the problems.

The responsibility of the body is on oneself. You cannot abstain yourself from the responsibility of the body requirements. The person must think of the health of the body and must take control of it before the diseases conquer it.

1

The Need of Good Health

There is always a need for good health; a person without the optimal health will be prone to more diseases and an unhealthy lifestyle. The good nutritional status of the body is important as it is vital and helpful to maintain all the important and essential functions of the body. The people who have maintained their body health are so good at growing and developing properly, and it will lead to the healthy as well as an active lifestyle.

The nutritional status of the body is the condition where the results of the nutrient content of the food effects the body and it is dependent on the content of the food that what is the relation of the nutrition needs to the body and it can make the body digest, absorb as well as use those nutrients.

When we want to have a good status regarding the nutrition, there are some essential conditions needed. The body always requires having enough and adequate nutrition as well as the safe food must be provided to eat. The body wants to have clean water, clean living conditions as well as the good sanitations. The human wants to have access to the good health services so that the information and knowledge about the essential nutrients must be provided. The person needs to have proper information as it is its ability to feed and care for the body and make it safer from any of the diseases or issues regarding the body. Every condition that has been discussed is good for the nutritional conditions and status, and they are usually affecting each other. If the nutrition is not focused, the results can be adverse. The person can face any particular diseases as well as the malnutrition.

Food

The good nutritional status is the reason behind the good physical health of a person. The nutritional status of the body has a direct impact of the foods that we consume and eat because of their nutritional and elemental composition. The content of the food is very important as it must have the essential elements that make the food able to provide the body with the contented feed. The good nutrition is relying on the right content and amount of the food. It is considered to be safe when we eat about the good quality of food that will later meet the nutritional needs of the body. The nutrition of body is fulfilling the body requirements of the elements. Here is the elemental composition list of the body is giving with the weight that tells that how the body is composed and what are the particular elements that are needed to the body to work correctly.

Elemental composition list

Element	*Composition in Grams*
Oxygen	43
Carbon	16
Hydrogen	7
Nitrogen	1.8
Calcium	1.0
Phosphorus	0.78
Potassium	0.14
Sulfur	0.14
Sodium	0.10
Chlorine	0.095
Magnesium	0.019
Iron*	0.0042

Fluorine	0.0026
Zinc	0.0023
Silicon	0.0010
Rubidium	0.00068
Strontium	0.00032
Bromine	0.00026
Lead	0.00012
Copper	0.000072
Aluminum	0.000060
Cadmium	0.000050
Cerium	0.000040
Barium	0.000022
Tin	0.000020
Iodine	0.000020
Titanium	0.000020
Boron	0.000018
Selenium	0.000015
Nickel	0.000015
Chromium	0.000014
Manganese	0.000012

Arsenic	0.000007
Lithium	0.000007
Mercury	0.000006
Cesium	0.000006
Molybdenum	0.000005
Germanium	5×10^{-6}
Cobalt	0.000003
Antimony	0.000002
Silver	0.000002
Niobium	0.0000015
Zirconium	0.000001
Lanthanum	8×10^{-7}
Tellurium	7×10^{-7}
Gallium	7×10^{-7}
Yttrium	6×10^{-7}
Bismuth	5×10^{-7}
Thallium	5×10^{-7}
Indium	4×10^{-7}
Gold	2×10^{-7}
Scandium	2×10^{-7}
Tantalum	2×10^{-7}

Vanadium	$1.1×10{-7}$
Thorium	$1×10{-7}$
Uranium	$1×10{-7}$
Samarium	$5.0×10{-8}$
Tungsten	$2.0×10{-8}$
Beryllium	$3.6×10{-8}$
Radium	$3×10{-14}$

*Iron = ~3 g in men, ~2.3 g in women

Food provides the basic energy to the body that is needed to have a healthy lifestyle. It gives the basic nutrients that help the body to perform all the functions required; it maintains the good health as well as it able to carry out the daily activities of life. The food we intake, have different ingredients, that are also known as the nutrients. These nutrients help the body to perform its activities well.

The food is made up of different ingredients. It is the complex composition of the nutrients that provide the essential elements to the body. Most of the nutrients that the body required cannot be produced by the human body itself. You need to take the adequate amounts of food that can fulfill the nutrition. It will make the body healthy, and diseases will be reduced and mitigated. The single type of food must not have all the nutritious elements required by the body. One type of food might have a higher level of particular elements while the other lacks in that particular element. The nutrients vary in each type of the food so that the person must make sure that all the food taken can provide with the minimum nutrients and elements required by the body. It is needed for good health as well as the nutritional status.

The people always try that they must get the food that is complete the requirements of the body and are well-nourished. It will help the people to grow, hunt or catch the food that they require. The people who can do it must have enough money to buy themselves food. The food you are buying must be safe, and healthy. It must not be contaminated so that body can react negatively.

MSM – Background

The MSM is also known as the Methyl Sulfonyl Methane (Dimethyl Sulfone). It is a nonmetallic as well a sulfur compound that is widely found in nature and used for various purposes. Sulfur is a material with a yellow appearance that has a different and various physical forms. It is found in the crystalline as well as the physical forms. It is the most important and the common substance that the body needs and it is found in the body. The sulfur is the element that completes the nutritional and elemental composition of the body that makes the body healthy. The sulfur plays an important role and character that helps in the nutrition of the human body. It is a very common fact the people usually overlook that. It is one of a compound that the body needs but the common people are not aware of it.

The MSM is a derivative of the DMSO. It is the abbreviation of the Dimethyl-sulfoxide. DMSO is a component that has been widely used in the treatments of the animals. It is usually helpful in treating the animals like horses. It is the element that will help to reduce the inflammation in the joints as well as the injured areas of the body. The smell and the impurities are the side effects that are usually limited to the humans for its widespread use.

The MSM is a compound that is usually appearing in white and crystallized form. The compound is odorless as well as it resembles the sugar. The sulfur component in the MSM compound makes up to 34% of it by weight. The MSM is known to be the richest compound in the context of the sulfur. The people who want to have the maximum sulfur can go for the MSM that completes the missing link of the human body's optimal health. MSM is the compound that is bitter in taste but slightly as well as it mixes with the water easily or in the juice. The solubility of the MSM is extremely high, and it is basic for the health of a person as the water and salt are the basic elements required by the body. It is not contaminated or toxic to the body but as safe as the water is to the body.

The MSM is the compound that belongs to the same elemental family that comprises of the oxygen. For the living things, the oxygen is very important in the environment, and they cannot live without it. The sulfur in the nutrition of the body replaces the oxygen when the body needs the source of the chemical energy essential for the life driving.

Made in the Clouds

The sulfur is important for the body, and it is required to fulfill the demands of the healthy body. The sources must be known from where the sulfur can be getting to fulfill the body requirements. Where the sulfur is made and how it can be utilized are the main questions that are asked when the person knows how important sulfur is to the body. The sulfur is an element that is present in the cells of the plants as well as the animals. When the plants and animals need the sulfur to use it for their bodies, they require it in the bio-available form. The sources of the sulfur must be clear as being the important and the essential element of the body; all the information must be focused. The people look forward to knowing how they can get the complete nutritional elements of their body. Their focus is on the sources that are easily available and accessible to not to compromise on the health of their bodies.

3

Major Responsibilities of Sulfur in the Body

—❦—

Here are some of the functions that are described in the book to tell that the sulfur is essential to carry the balanced activities and maintain these functions properly. There are important and major responsibilities of the body that must be carried by the involvement of the sulfur. These important functions are not possible without the sulfur and its compounds. The people who make use of the sulfur and maintain the minimum level of the body will provide better health and reduce the dis-functionality of the body.

The three important roles of the body that makes use of the sulfur are described. They are important functions that can create issues for the body if not maintained.

Dehydration and Detoxification

The element, sulfur is very important for the ionic exchange. It has a particular responsibility towards the ionic exchange of the sodium-potassium pump in the body cells. The sulfur is an essential element in the body. It is needed for the maintenance of the permeability of the cell membrane. The people who look forward to the maintenance levels of the sulfur in the body will make sure that they body will provide the essential nutrients to these activities. The nutrients and the elements are taken to the cells and the toxic materials as well as the waste products of the cells can be excreted out. This is the phenomenon of the dehydration as well as the detoxification.

These are the two functions that are important for the health. If the body is always dehydrated and the entire water component is excreted out, it will not function properly. The maintenance of the health is achieved when the dehydration is coped out. The body must not reach the levels of the dehydration. Those who are always dehydrated cannot function properly, and their lifestyle is affected. The detoxification is important for the body. The toxins and the toxic materials of the body must be excreted out so that the healthy thing replaces them. The people who have been contaminated with the toxins do not function properly.

Energy

Energy is important for the body to keep the balance in the healthy lifestyle. The human body cannot work if it does not have the proper levels of the energy. the energy levels are drained out once the body does not meet the nutritional and elemental levels required by the body. The body needs proper food and diet that help them to get the proper elements required to charge the energy levels. Sulfur is the element that is most important contribution towards the energy. The sulfur is an important component of the insulin. It is an important and significant hormone that is essential for the regulation of the glucose. The regulation of the sulfur levels wills uptake the glucose by cells for the use in the body as the energy. The energy is maintained when the sulfur is maintained. They are directly responsible and dependent on their functions. The sulfur is also important for the thiamine and biotin. These are needed for the body when the carbohydrate metabolism has to be undertaken.

The body functions are not possible without the essential elements. Whether the sulfur does not have direct contact with the function but the proper functionality can be achieved just through the sulfur and its presence in the body.

Structure and Function

The sulfur is an essential element. It is required by the body when the proper functionality has to be achieved. The sulfur is the component that makes up the protein, and then the protein has been used to make up the body tissues. The most body tissues like the skin, organs, blood vessels, nails and hair, are made of the protein. When all these parts of the body require sulfur, how it can be out looked. The sulfur is the element that is making up the flexible and elastic S-S bonds in the protein that provide the elasticity and the flexibility of the movement of the body and its parts. The sulfur can repair and heal the tissues that have been damaged or destroyed by the aging, free radical attack as well as due to the injuries. The cells in the body are always in the state of regeneration. They are found to regenerating at different rates, but they are always changing and replacing the body parts.

Rate of the Cellular Removal

When all the cells are regenerating with a different pace, here are the examples that will tell the fastest to the slowest rate in which it has been carrying out the regeneration.

Epithelial Cells: It is the important part of the skin. It makes up those tissues that cover the whole body in the name of the skin. It constitutes the line of the digestive, urinary as well as the respiratory tracts. These are the fastest removing cells as you know that the skin is the outer layer of the body. It keeps removing the cells in the form of the dead skin where the friction is more. So the regeneration of the new cells takes the place of old ones at a faster pace.

Connective Tissue: The connective tissues of the body are very important. And the sulfur has been used to regenerate them but at a medium pace. These connective tissues include the cells of fats, fibrous cartilage, and the mucopolysaccharides. These are the points that help the maintenance of the elasticity as well as well the flexibility of the body. It is the component that holds the body together. The connective tissues have great importance in the body as it is the important component of the organs of the body.

Muscle, Bone Cells, and Nervous Cells: these are the slowest regenerating parts of the body. The regeneration is the slowest, so the sulfur is needed for the cells of the above two parts of the body. The body might take up to seven to eight years while replacing the cells. These are not considered to be sulfur needed areas as the minimum quantity of sulfur element is required in this part of the body.

4
Sulfur Deficiency

Most of the people are sulfur deficient. Are you sulfur deficient? You must ask this question to you. You must keep checking the body and its regulations. The body needs proper diet. The diet that has the essential and necessary components will achieve the status of the nutritional diet. The food must contain all the essential elements required by the body. When the person looks forward to get all the elements from food, he must think that not all kinds of food have all the elements. There must be a combination of food and diet that can help the body to achieve the nutritional elements for the body that are required to the body.

The deficiency of the sulfur in the body can cause various effects. These might include the different ones that make the body associated with further issues. The people who lack in the sulfur elements can face;

- Healing of the wounds but slowly, it is because the cells are not regenerated at a lower rate.
- The scar tissues can be found, and the skin is usually damaged.
- The nails are brittle as well as the hair is brittle.

- There are problems related to the gastro intestines.
- The inflammation of the cells is unregulated.
- There is dysfunction of the lungs and the respiratory system.
- The problems are associated with the immune system.
- Arthritis issues are common.
- The people are more prone to acne.
- There are rashes over the skin.
- The people can face depression and stress regularly.
- Losing memory is a common effect.

The MSM supplement is very important as it will give adequate organic sources to the body for its use towards the particular areas. The body requires the MSM as it is needed to overcome the deficiency that is prominent to all the issues discussed before. The body is constantly repairing itself, but when the body is not provided with the essential elements, the outcome will not be perfect and irregular.

The medical sciences have investigated that the body that is deficient in the MSM do not have a particular link towards the optimal health. This type of body will be prone to arthritis. There is a relation when the MSM is deficient, the particular diseases like allergies, Alzheimer's diseases as well as asthma. It is also associated with the dermatological issues, periodontal situations as well as cancer.

5
Sources of Sulfur

The existence of the processed foods had created many issues as when the foods were organic and raw, the sources of MSM and sulfur were straight and common. The MSM was naturally found, and it was easy to obtain from the particular foods. The sulfur is the natural component that is available and easy to get from the foods. The sulfur in the soil is very important. The sulfur in the soil is varying with the greater amount, and it is also getting deficient with the time. When the soil is deficient, the crop will not have a particular amount of sulfur that will be further consumed. The processed foods and even the natural foods are still deficient in the sulfur.

The foods that are properly produced can have sufficient amount of sulfur that will be further consumed from the foods.

Foods that have Sulfur

- The fresh fruits are important as they are having the greatest amount of the sulfur.

- The fresh vegetables that are produced in the soil that has essential elements in it will contain the increased amount of sulfur.
- Dried beans including the Soybeans
- Fish in addition to Seafood
- The meat in the form of beef and mutton or the chicken or fish.
- Eggs that have properties of protein as well contain sulfur.
- Milk, cheese and other dairy products.
- Tea and coffee
- Chocolates
- Garlic as well as the onions
- The herb named as the Horsetail
- Wheat germ and Amino Acids

What Sulfur can do?

The sulfur is an important consideration for the body. It can be sourced out from various points. It is needed for the body, and it can do wonders. The people who use sulfur are the ones that enjoy its wonders. There are different benefits of sulfur to your body.

1. Sulfur is important, and it is the third most abundant element that is found in the body. It is mostly concentrated in the muscles, bones, and skin of the person and it is an essential element. The sulfur creates amino acids that are used to create proteins needed in the production of the hormones, enzymes, antibodies as well as the proteins. The body uses the sulfur and stores it daily that is needed to get optimal health and

nutrition.

2. The sulfur is needed for the production of the insulin. It is used for the metabolism of the carbohydrate, but when it is deficient, the pancreas is not able to produce the insulin needed to make energy from the glucose levels.

3. Sulfur is used for the detoxification of the cells in the body, and it reduces the inflammation and pain. The health of the cells is very important as it increases the absorption of the nutrients while the toxins and wastes are released.

4. The hardening of the arteries and veins are reduced with the help of the sulfur as it increases the flexibility and elasticity. It makes the arteries breathable.

5. The element of sulfur is possibly called the beauty mineral as it keeps the complexion of the body clear, as well as the hairs, become smooth and less brittle.

6. The soil absorbs the sulfur from the rainwater and seawater. The natural cycle has been made that helps the plants to get the sulfur from the soil or nature and then the humans consume it through the plants and animals.

7. The people used to consume the organic food but now processed foods have replaced them that make it less possible to achieve the sulfur.

8. The MSM has the properties of the anti-parasitic actions as well as the anti-allergic. These are considered to do wonders to the immune system of the body.

9. The vitamin C and MSM of the body are the best combinations that is helpful towards the body and its production of the cells as well as the connective tissue. The vitamin C can support the healthy regeneration of the cells.

6

MSM – The Missing Link to Optimal Health

The MSM is the only way that can be the reason to complete the missing link to the optimal health of the person. The health is very important, and it can be improved through the MSM. The MSM is recommended to those who have been appreciating good health. The sports enthusiasts, as well as the athletes, make use of the MSM to speed up the recovery of the consequences of the workouts as well as the improvement of the performance. The people who are having the degenerative diseases use the MSM to cure themselves. The MSM is the base that can be used to maintain the healthy lifestyle, get a balanced diet, improving the health and quality of life as well as the getting the cure for different problems.

It is used to be a supplement that was taken from the organic food and the diet but nowadays the food is not able to provide these supplements. The elements of sulfur are not available on the plants as the crops are deficient in the sulfur. The cycle where the sulfur has to be in concentration is decreased. The MSM is the compound that is now being produced artificially. The people can undertake these supplements to overcome the deficiencies that have been produced in their bodies. The MSM is the source of energy to the body, and it facilitates the body in concern that the body will be able to get the essential tools that will cure the problems. The vitality of the body will be maintained through it.

7

How Safe is MSM?

The MSM is just as similar in toxicity as you can find the toxicity in the water. When the experiments were taken out by the medical sciences, the people were given a dosage of the MSM, 1 gram per kg of the body weight for about 30 days; there were no negative and toxic effects were seen on the body. More than 12000 patients were given MSM in the case of their treatments, and they were seen with positive results later on.

8
Conclusion

The sulfur is important for the body, and when you cannot consume it through the organic food or in the food intake, you have to take MSM orally that is made artificially in the labs. The MSM has a huge amount of sulfur in it that is important for the health. It is taken according to the body weight of the person. The people who cannot get the sulfur through their diet must ensure themselves to take it. They are an important element to the body that is why it is essential to consume it regularly and restrict the ability of the body to get the diseases.

The missing link to the optimal health is only filled and completed through the intake of the MSM; these can be taken from artificial or natural sources. The recommendation is to take naturally, but there is no problem if the intake can be through artificial means. The people must make sure that the sulfur need in the body is fulfilled anybody issues can be reduced to it. The complete nutrition including the sulfur can achieve the optimal health and a healthy lifestyle.

Disclaimer

Introduction

By using this book, you accept this disclaimer in full.

No advice

The book contains information. The information is not advice, and should not be treated as such.

If you think you may be suffering from any medical condition you should seek immediate medical attention. You should never delay seeking medical advice, disregard medical advice, or discontinue medical treatment because of information in the book.

No representations or warranties

To the maximum extent permitted by applicable law and subject to section below, we exclude all representations, warranties, undertakings and guarantees relating to the book.

Without prejudice to the generality of the foregoing paragraph, we do not represent, warrant, undertake or guarantee:

- that the information in the book is correct, accurate, complete or non-misleading;

- that the use of the guidance in the book will lead to any particular outcome or result.

Limitations and exclusions of liability

The limitations and exclusions of liability set out in this section and elsewhere in this disclaimer: are subject to section 6 below; and govern all liabilities arising under the disclaimer or in relation to the book, including liabilities arising in contract, in tort (including negligence) and for breach of statutory duty.

We will not be liable to you in respect of any losses arising out of any event or events beyond our reasonable control.

We will not be liable to you in respect of any business losses, including without limitation loss of or damage to profits, income, revenue, use, production, anticipated savings, business, contracts, commercial opportunities or goodwill.

We will not be liable to you in respect of any loss or corruption of any data, database or software.

We will not be liable to you in respect of any special, indirect or consequential loss or damage.

Exceptions

Nothing in this disclaimer shall: limit or exclude our liability for death or personal injury resulting from negligence; limit or exclude our liability for fraud or fraudulent misrepresentation; limit any of our liabilities in any way that is not permitted under applicable law; or exclude any of our liabilities that may not be excluded under applicable law.

Severability

If a section of this disclaimer is determined by any court or other competent authority to be unlawful and/or unenforceable, the other sections of this disclaimer continue in effect.

If any unlawful and/or unenforceable section would be lawful or enforceable if part of it were deleted, that part will be deemed to be deleted, and the rest of the section will continue in effect.

Law and jurisdiction

This disclaimer will be governed by and construed in accordance with Swiss law, and any disputes relating to this disclaimer will be subject to the exclusive jurisdiction of the courts of Switzerland.